# PATANJALI YOGA SUTRAS

## IN THE LIGHT OF KRIYA

**LAHIRI MAHASAYA**



SANAGE
PUBLISHING HOUSE

Paperback: 978-811909036-5



Printed by:

Sanage Publishing House LLP
Mumbai, India

sanagepublishing@gmail.com

**Shyama Charan Lahiri** (30 September 1828 - 26 September 1895), best known as **Lahiri Mahasaya**, was an Indian yogi guru who founded the Kriya Yoga school. In 1861, his non-physical master Mahavatar Babaji appeared to him, ordering him to revive the yogic science of Kriya Yoga to the public after centuries of its guarding by masters.

He became known in the West through Paramahansa Yogananda, a disciple of Sri Yukteswar Giri, and through Yogananda's 1946 book Autobiography of a Yogi, considering him a Yogavatar, or "Incarnation of Yoga," since Lahiri himself was chosen by the yogic masters to disseminate the principles of yoga to the world.

# List of Chapters

# Chapter 1

# Samadhi Pada : Meditation

### *1*
### *Atha Yoganusasana.*

Now the discourse on Yoga begins.

Whatever state of attunement is attained by dissolving the intellect, or thoughts, fixing the mind on the *Kutastha Bindu*, or "the divine spot", continuously looking at one Star like a fool is called *Samadhi.*

When that state is not free from reasoning, it is called *Sampragnat Samadhi*, and when it is free from reasoning, it is called *Asampragnat Samadhi.*

### *2*
### *Yogaschittvavritti nirodha.*

When the *Vrittis*, or "the waves" of the China, "the heart," are automatically dissolved, this is the state of *Yoga.*

*3*

***Tada drastu swarupe abasthanam.***

Then the Consciousness is automatically seen. In that state of *Samadhi*, the seer is in his Self, or he is established in Consciousness.

*4*

***Vrittiswarupyamitaratra.***

In any state other than *Samadhi*, the Self is experienced according to the waves of the heart.

When the seer's reflection falls on the surface of the trembling water of a lake, it appears as though he were seeing but not experiencing who he is.

Due to the restlessness of the water, the reflection always takes on different shapes as though the seer himself were taking on different shapes.

Likewise in any state other than Samadhi, the restlessness of the heart appears to be the restlessness of the Self.

*5*

***Vrittvaya panchatajya klistayaklista.***

There are five kinds of *Vrittis*, or "waves", irrespective of being attached to or detached from worldly affairs. and they are centered around attachment due to pleasure and detachment due to suffering.

*6*

***Pramanabiparjyaya bikalpa nidrasmrittaya.***

Proof, confusion, alternatives, sleep, and remembrance. These are the five kinds of waves.

*7*

***Tatra prataksyanumanagama Pramanani.***

Perception inference and outwardness, that is, experiencing with the senses, are proofs.

*8*

***Biparjyo mithyajnanamatatadrupa pratisdtham.***

When the unreal is taken for the Real, this is called confusion, the opposite awareness.

*9*

***Sabdajnananupati bastusunyo bikalpa.***

Knowledge gained from words is accordingly experienced, in other words, they are only an alternative, or imagination. But the real thing is Void.

*10*

***Abhabapratyayalambana vrittvinidra.***

The ceasing of external awareness of sensations is called sleep. Although there is no awareness of things in sleep, still they are felt.

*11*

***Anubhuta bisayasampramosa smroti.***

Trying to reproduce previous experience is remembrance.

*12*

***Avyasa baoiragyabhyang tannirodha.***

Only by *Practice* and *Renunciation* can one stop those waves of the heart.

*13*

***Tatra sthito jatnayabhyasa.***

What is practice?
Holding onto the *Kutastha* with efforts to keep the mind tranquil is practice.

*14*

***Satu dirghakalanorantajya satkarasebito drirabhumi.***

Continuous Kriya practice will stabilize that practice.

*15*

***Dristanusrabikabisaya bitrisnasya basikarasangjnya boragyam.***

Renunciation is the giving up of all desires seen and unseen and of what is heard but not seen when the seeker remains attuned in *Samadhi.*

***16***

***Tatparang purusakhyatergunaboitrisnasyam.***

Thereafter, having seen the mysterious supreme Being, remaining attuned in that state, the seeker develops disinterest towards qualities.

***17***

***Bitarka vicharanandasmita rupanugamat samprajnat.***

*Sampragnat Samadhi* takes place due to arguments,reasoning, Bliss, the subtle way of awareness in the subtle atom, and seeing Oneself. There are four kinds of *Samadhi*:

1. Argumentative (*Savitarka*): Is whatever I have seen so?
2. Reasoning (*Savichara*): Is what I have seen disillusionment from *Maya*?
3. Bliss (*Sananda*): Only to have Bliss.
4. Subtle (*Asmita*): Seeing in disembodiment.

*18*

***Biram pratyayabhyasapurba sangsakarasesoyanya.***

Continuous practice of restraint: *Sampragnat Samadhi*, or "the unconsolidated state of Samadhi" eventually finds its consolidated state, which is called *Asampragnat Samadhi.*

*19*

***Bhabapratyayo bidehaprakritilayanam.***

The Knowledge attained due to the dissolution of the sense of body, ego, and also Nature is the cause of *Samadhi.* The practice of tranquil air by one whose heart is dissolved in Nature stabilizes the heart only until reappearance.

*20*

***Sraddhaviryasmritisamadhi prajnapurbak itaresam.***

Others attain *Samadhi* with *Sraddha*, or "reverence," *Virya*, or "inwardness," *Smriti*, or "regeneration," Yoga *Samadhi*, or "Attunement," and Wisdom.

Reverence is generated by the practice of Kriya.

Similarly, inwardness and regeneration provide universal intellect resulting in unconsolidated *(Sampragnat) Samadhi.*

Continuous practice thereafter generates Renunciation resulting in the consolidated state, or *Asampragnat Samadhi.*

***21***

***Tibrasangbeganamasanna.***

By determined meditation *Samadhi* is achieved sooner.

***22***

***Mridumadhyadhimatratvattatoyapi bisesa.***

There are gradations: mild, middle and intensive.

***23***

***Iswarapranidhanatba.***

By holding onto the inner Self with exclusive devotion, one can attain *Samadhi.*

***24***

***Klesakarmabipakasayorparamrista Purusabisesa Iswara.***

*Kutastha*, the inner Self, is above suffering and the results of good and bad actions.

***25***

***Tatra niratisayang sarbajnabijam.***

That inner Self possesses the seed of Omniscience, that is, holding onto Him, Omniscience is generated. It is called stabilization.

## *26*

***Sa eba purbesamapi Guru kalenanabachhedat.***

That inner Self is beyond time, therefore, greater than *Brahma*, or "the Creator".

## *27*

***Tasya vachaka Pranaba.***

*Pranaba* is the representative of the same, *OM*. As the burning flame is revealed automatically, likewise, in the state of *Samadhi*, the sound of *OM* is heard spontaneously.

## *28*

***Tajjapaastadarthabhabanam.***

The seeker will think that sound of *OM* to be God, or *Iswara*. Listening to *OM* is God.

## *29*

***Tata pratyakchetanadhigamoyapyan-tararayabhabascha.***

Then every step provides the knowledge of *Iswara*, or God and will be the obstruction to attachments of the heart.

*30*

***Byadhistyanasangsayapramadalasyabirati brantidarsanalabddhabhumi katvanabasthitatvani chittvabikshepasteyantaraya.***

The following are the means of distraction for the heart of a Yogi, which make his attention outward:

1. Disease : Disharmony of breath.

2. Ineffectiveness of the heart.

3. Doubts.

4. Wrong conceptions.

5. Lethargy : Unwillingness to practice Yoga due to bodily awareness and heaviness of heart.

6. Unawareness of the heart specifically.

7. Wrong Observation.

8. Absence of the ground of *Samadhi*.

9. Inability to stabilize, even after obtaining the ground of *Samadhi*.

*31*

***Dukhadormanasyangmejayatva swasa praswasa bikshepasahyabhuba.***

Suffering is threefold, namely spiritual, cosmic and material.

Restlessness of heart and disharmony of breath are the causes of distraction of the Tranquil Heart. Transcending them, abandoning expectations for results thereof, the seeker should enter into *Samadhi.*

*32*

***Tatpratisedhakarthamekatattvabhyasa.***

To remove those obstructions, one must start practicing to make the mind one-pointed.

*33*

***Moitrikarunamuditopekshanang sukhadukhapunyapunyabisayanang bhabanataschittaprasadanam.***

In place of pleasure and pain, right and wrong, friendship, kindness, contentment and indifference are to be developed. That is, in place of happiness, friendship; of pain, kindness; of righteousness, contentment; and of wrong, indifference.

These are to be cultivated with contemplative heart, holding onto the Self.

It usually provides satisfaction.

*34*

***Prachhardanabidharanabhyang ba Pranasya.***

Also, by the practice of *Pranayam*, the waves of the heart becomes tranquil.

**Prachhardhan** : Extracting air through the nose from the stomach, that is, inhaling, and

**Bidharan** : Exhaling.

### *35*

***Bisayavati ba pravrittvirutpanna manasa sthiti nibandhan.***

Even tendencies towards objects produced in the mind by the senses, that is, the knowledge of divine smell and divine taste, arise, and the waves of the heart become tranquil.

### *36*

***Bisoka ba jyotismati.***

All is beyond objects, that is, the Atom of *Brahma*, or the ultimate Self.

This inner Wisdom is called *Bisoka (Asmita)*. This is Illumination.

The Yogis attain the state of Tranquility.

### *37*

***Bitaragabisayang ba chittam.***

Even by being disinterested in the objects, the Yogi attains the tranquil state. Simply by turning away from the world, that is, by making himself inwards, the Yogi realizes the Self or who he is.

*38*
***Swapnanidrajnanalambanamba.***

Even by the means of dreams and drowsy feelings, it can be attained.

The seeker can realize the Self even through the divine grace of dreams and drowsy feelings.

*39*
***Jathabhimatadhyanatba.***

By whatever means, if the waves are tranquil, that will bring inner Realization.

*40*
***Paramanu paramamahattvantoyasyabasikara.***

Thus the Yogi controls the Atom and the Complete Whole. Now, the tranquil heart is being described.

*41*
***Tatsatha tadanjanata samapattvi.***

The restrained heart, the person of the renunciated heart, whether concentrating on the senses, on the Self, or on Oneness finds the same result eventually.

As the marble stone absorbs the color of the diamond when it is near, similarly, for the realized Yogi the whole manifested World is colored as the Self and he becomes free.

When the heart is established in that state of the Self, the heart becomes One with the Self.

*42*

***Tatra sabdarthajnanabikalpoi sankirna sabitarka samapattvi.***

By means of sound, meaning, knowledge and rejection, *Savitarka Samadhi* is held which is very narrow.

Gradually greater *Nirvitarka Samadhi* is held, which is being described.

*43*

***Smritiparisudho swarupasunyevarthamatranirbhasa nivitarka.***

When remembrance is purified, then *Nirvitarka Samadhi* is held. In such a state, objects only appear as Void.

*44*

***Etayoirba savichara nirvichara cha suksma bisaya byakhyata.***

By *Savitarka*, that is, Argument, and *Nirvitarka*, that is, being free from argument, both gross and subtle things are explained.

*45*

***Suksmabisayatvanchalinga parjabasan.***

What is subtle? The objects of the subtle way are:

- the atom of the smell of earth,
- the atom of the taste of water,
- the atom of the sight of fire,
- the atom of the touch of air, and
- the atom of the hearing of ether.

Among them, the Sign is subtle, and the Signless is more subtle.

After the signless, there is no subtlety; therefore, subtlety is the gist, and the supreme Person is subtle.

### *46*

### ***Ta eba sajiva samadhi.***

The four kinds of *Samadhi* with seed are: *Savitarka, Nirvitarka, Savichara*, and *Nirvichara.*

There are different types of *Samadhi*, or Attunements, depending on the position of the intellect, namely:

1. *Savitarka* (argumentative),
2. *Nivitarka* (being free from argument),
3. *Savichara* (with reasoning), and
4. *Nirvichara* (free from reasoning).

All these types involve the seed of the intellect.

*47*

***Nirvicharaboisaradyayadhyatmapraada.***

The grace of the Self is attained through the pure *Nirvichara* (perfectly free from reasoning, or thoughts.)

*48*

***Ritambhara tatra Prajna.***

In this state, wisdom finds its Realization. When the intellect is dissolved, everything is known perfectly.

*49*

***Srutanumanaprajnabhyamanyabisaya bisesarthatvat.***

Wisdom blessed by the grace of the Self is different from wisdom resulting from words and inference.

*50*

***Tajja sangskaroyanyasangskara pratibandhi.***

When attunement in inner Wisdom is achieved through *Samadhi*, then attention cannot go outward.

*51*

***Tasyapi nirodhe sarbanirodhannirbija samadhi.***

Gradually inward attention is dissolved in the Self and thereby the *Nirbija Samadhi*, or the Perfect state, is achieved.

In other words, when there is no *Sanskaras*, or innate awareness, then the seeking self establishes himself in the ultimate Self.

This is called pure Liberation.

# Chapter 2

# Sadhana Pada : Procedure

*1*

***Tapaswadhyayeswara pranidhanani kriya yoga.***

Now, we turn to the instruction of how to practice Yoga, which is to be practiced under the direct guidance of the *Guru*, i.e., *Kutastha*.

*Tapa, Swadhyaya* and *Iswarapranidhana* constitute Kriya Yoga:

1. *Tapa* : *Pranaba*, or *OM*, which is spontaneously heard.

2. *Swadhyaya* : The chanting of *OM*.

3. *Iswarapranidhana* : Holding onto the Self, surrendering all actions to the Self and offering inner Realization; all of which are done by Him.

*2*

***Sa hi kriyayoga samadhibhabanartha klesatanu karanarthacha.***

To remove suffering and to attain *Samadhi*, Kriya Yoga must be practiced.

The holding onto *Samadhi* by means of practicing Kriya removes suffering of the body and mind.

Gradually, *Nada*, or the inner Sound, is heard, leaving no room for all imagination and thoughts of the mind.

Afterwards, the supreme Being and inner Wisdom are both attained.

*3*

***Abidyasmitaragadwesavinibesa panchaklesa.***

There are the five sufferings:

1. *Avidya* (ignorance),
2. *Asmita* (egoism),
3. *Raga* (attachment),
4. *Dwesa* (hatred), and
5. *Avinibesa*, (attachment to the body).

*4*

***Abidyakshetramuttaresang prasuptatanubichhhinnodaram.***

Ignorance is the root of all other sufferings.

Attachment and hatred, whichever form they may take, be the weak or scattered or indifferent, are due to ignorance.

*5*

***Anityasuchidukhanatmasu nityasuchisukhatmakhyatir abidya.***

One's understanding, eternal in the transient, pure in the impure, happiness in the unhappiness, and the Self in the not-self is ignorance.

*6*

***Drigdarasaktyorekatmatebayasmita.***

When there is a seer and seen experiencing Oneness, this is called *Asmita*. That is, when the egoism of the seeker who does not realize the supreme Self to be within himself as Seer erroneously confuses the supreme Self with the senses, this is called *Asmita*.

*7*

***Sukhanusayi raga.***

Attachment is developed in happiness.

*8*

***Dukhanusayi dwesa.***

Anger arising from sorrow is called *Dwes*, or violence and hatred.

*9*

***Swarasabahi bidusoyapi tatharudoyang avinibesa.***

When a man of Knowledge who knows that birth and death involve sorrow still develops the tendency for attachment, this is called *avinibesa.*

*10*

***Te pratiprasabaheya sukshma.***

The subtle five means of suffering should be destroyed by burning the seeds. Thereby, one goes to *Brahma*, or the ultimate Self.

*11*

***Dhyanaheyastadvrittaya.***

The means of destroying the gross form of the *Vrittis*, or waves of attachment, is described.

The mind of one who holds onto the Self in meditation does not go to *Vrittis*, or waves of attachments.

*12*

***Klesamula karmasayodristadristajanmabedaniya.***

The known (seen) actions of this life and the deposit of unseen actions of past lives are the causes for attachment, anger, etc.

*13*

***Sati mule tadbipako jatyayurbhoga.***

In fact, this deposit of sufferings determines the longevity and nature of pleasure and pain.

*14*

***Te haladaparitapaphala punyapunyahetutvang.***

Pleasure and pain depend on the nature of righteous and wrong actions accordingly. Righteous action results in happiness while wrong action results in suffering.

*15*

***Parinamatapasangskaradukhoigunavrittvibirodhachha dukhameba sarbang vivekina.***

But the man of Knowledge considers all states of manifestation to be sorrow due to the influence of Nature born qualities.

*16*

***Heya dukhamanagatam.***

The predestined sorrows are considered as indispensable by the Yogi.

*17*

***Drastri drsyayo sangjogo heyehetu.***

The consciousness of the seer and the intellect of the seen, when associated, become the cause of suffering. Once removed, suffering does not continue.

The cause of suffering is outward attention with attachments. When the seeker makes himself inward from the outward attentions, then the cause of suffering is removed.

## *18*

***Prakasa kriyasthiti silambhutendriy atmakambhog apabargarthang dasyam.***

What is seen?
The following are seen:

- *Sattva* (illumination),
- *Raja* (active),
- *Tama* (inactive),
- *Bhutas* (beings),
- *Indriyas* (sensations),
- *Pravrittvi* (attachments), and
- *Nivrittvi* (restraint).

## *19*

***Bisesabisesa lingamatralingani gunaparbani.***

These are the different states of qualities:

- *Bises* (comprehensive),
- *Abises* (incomprehensive),
- *Linga Matra* (the first state of manifestation), and
- *Alinga* (the last state of quality is signless or invisible).

*Bises*, or comprehensive: the five elements including the Sky.

*Abises*, or incomprehensive: Sound and the subtle five elements, etc.

*Linga Matra*, or the first state of manifestation: *Mahattattva*, or the cosmic state.

*Alinga*, or signless: the super-subtle state.

Afterwards (in the next verse), the seer is described.

### *20*

***Drastadrisimatra suddhoyapi pratyayanupasya.***

The Seer is Consciousness only. Purity is established in the absence of modifications, or manifestations, yet the subject is seer. The character of the seen which is seen by the seer depends on the search outwardly for the object by the seer's intellect, or *Buddhi*.

### *21*

***Tadartha eba drisyasyatma.***

What is the reflection between them?

The manifestation, or seen, is meant for the enjoyment of the seer.

*22*

***Kritarthampratinastamapyanastas-tadanyasadharanatvat.***

To a realized Yogi, these tricks of the mind, that is, the manifestation of the world, are destroyed, but for the ordinary people, they still exist.

Ordinary people do not see the hollowness of the world's appearance.

*23*

***Swa Swamisaktyo swarapopalabddhi hetu sangjoga.***

The association is to realize *Swa-Sakti*, or the nature of the seen, and *Swami-Sakti*, or the nature of the seer.

The seer and seen are associated as the sensor and the sensed.

The object of enjoyment, the enjoyer's enjoyment character and the enjoyment itself are without beginning.

This is the unreasonable association, or relation.

*24*

***Tasya heturheyamabidya.***

Therefore, ignorance must be destroyed.

Wiping out ignorance by destroying the ego is the only way to attain absolute Knowledge. The aim of practicing Yoga is to destroy the ego, or ignorance.

### *25*

***Tadbhabat sangjogabhabo hanantaddwase kaibalyam.***

Whenever Enlightenment begins due to the absence of ignorance, the absence of unreasonable association spontaneously takes place, and the destruction of such association is called *Kaibalya*, or eternal Realization.

### *26*

***Vivekakhyatirabiplabahanopaya.***

The means of that destruction is unceasing Enlightenment.

### *27*

***Tasua saptadha prantabhumi Prajna.***

When enlightenment starts, seven kinds of wisdoms are attained.

Action ceases by the following four state:

1. By the influence of Knowledge, generating the feeling to ignore future sufferings,

2. By restraint,

3. By *Samadhi*, or Attunement, and

4. By Wisdom.

And *Chitta*, the heart, becomes free from attachment by three stages:

1. The decrease and dissolution of mental qualities.

2. The destruction of the reappearance of the mental qualities due to the absence of the need for them.

3. Inner Realization of the supreme Being in the inner Light beyond all qualities.

### *28*

***Yoganganusthanada sudhvikshaye jnanadiptira viveka khtate.***

By the practice of the eightfold Yoga, impurities and qualities are purified to enrich righteousness, and inner Revelations begin.

### *29*

***Yamaniyamasan pranayama pratyahara dharana dhyana samadhayo yastangani.***

The following are the eight steps of Yoga:

1. *Yama* (restraint),

2. *Niyama* (rule),

3. *Asana* (steadfastness in sitting),
4. *Pranayam* (respiration),
5. *Pratyahar* (inwardness),
6. *Dharana* (glimpse of Tranquility),
7. *Dhyana* (meditation), and
8. *Samadhi* (Attunement).

### *30*

***Tatrahingsasatyasteyabrahmacharyapari-graha yama.***

The following points constitute *Yama*:

1. *Ahingsa* (nonviolence),
2. *Satya* (truth),
3. *Asteya* (non-stealing),
4. *Brahmacharaya* (celibacy, or restraining the senses to hold onto the Self), and
5. *Aparigraha* (not accepting help from others).

### *31*

***Jatidesakalasamayanbachhina sarbabhouma mahavratam.***

To remain steadfast to these vows in life, regardless of caste, nation, time and need, are universal vows.

*32*
***Socha santosa tapa swadhyayeswara pranidhanani niyama.***

The following points constitute *Niyama* (rule):

1. *Socha* (external purity)
2. *Santosa* (internal purity)
3. *Tapa* (that which can be known personally from the *Guru*)
4. *Swadhyaya* (listening to the sound of *OM*), and
5. *Pranidhana* (holding onto the Self).

*33*
***Etesang yamaniyamanang bitarkabadhane pratipaksha bhabanam.***

To remove doubts regarding *Yama* and *Niyama*, the cultivation of good sentiments is necessary.

*34*
***Bitarkahingsadaya kritakaritanumodita lobhakrodhamoha purbaka mridumadhyadhimatra dukhajnananatphala iti prati paksha bhabanam.***

The following brings infinite sufferings, sorrow and ignorance: violence done by a person himself or Commissioned by a person, greed, anger, attachment and death. The absence of these brings happiness.

***35***

***Ahingsa pratisthayang tat sannidho bairityaga.***

Enmity is dissolved in the man who is established in *Ahingsa*, or nonviolence.

***36***

***Satyapratisthayang kriyaphalasrayatvam.***

When *Satya*, or Truth is established, then *Kriya* becomes fruitful. Then without practicing Kriya, one enjoys the fruits of Kriya.

***37***

***Asteyapratisthayang sarbaratnopasthanam.***

When *Asteya* or non stealing, is established, then all things come before the Yogi.

***38***

***Brahmacharya praisthayang Viryulabha***

When *Brahmacharya*, or celibacy is established, then energy is generated. When one is established in the advice of the *Guru*, then one gets Realization.

*39*

***Aparigrahasthairye janmakathatsambodha***

In the establishment of *Aparigraha* or not taking any help from others, one knows what he was, what he will be, etc.

*40*

***Sochatswangjugupsa paroirasangsarga.***

When *Socha*, or purity, is established on account of feelings of impurity, one hates his own body and disassociates from others also.

*41*

***Kinchsatva suddhisoumanasoikagrendriyatmadarsana jogyatvanicha.***

From Purity are generated Divinity, Tranquility, concentration, mastery over the senses and the capacity for realizing the Self.

*42*

***Sontashadanuttam sukhalabha.***

By *Santosh*, or contentment, a great deal of happiness is achieved.

*43*

***Kayendriyasiddhirasuddhikshayattapasa.***

From *Tapa*, or the endurance of hardships and mastery over the senses, impurities are transcended.

By holding onto *Kutastha Brahma* according to advice of the *Guru*, the mind becomes pure, and afterwards such yogic powers are gained as making oneself small and hearing from far distances.

**44**
***Swadhyayadistadevatasamprayayoga.***

By *Swadhyaya*, or self-study, the *Istadev*, or the desired deity (the desired form of the Lord), is seen.

By hearing the sound of *OM* (inner Sound), gods, seers and realized ones are seen and in time, results are accrued.

**46**
***Samadhisiddhiriswarapranidhanat.***

By holding the mind steadfastly on the *Kutastha, Samadhi* and satisfaction of all sorts of desires are attained and the knowledge of faraway places, past and future is also achieved.

**46**
***Tatra sthirasukhamasanam.***

In whichever sitting position the mind remains tranquil and happiness is generated, that particular sitting position should be practiced. To remain steadfast, that *Asana*, or particular sitting position, is needed.

*47*

***Prajatnasoithilyanantyasamapattibhyam.***

Taking care of idleness and holding onto the infinite Self should be the seat of *Asana.*

*48*

***Tatodwandwanabhighat.***

By the establishment of such steadfastness, the seeker becomes free from hot and cold, thirst and hunger and the sense of dualism.

*49*

***Tasmin sati Swasa praswasayorgati bichheda Pranayama.***

When one has reached the steadfast sitting position, when inhaling and exhaling naturally stop, then *Pranayam* is held.

*50*

***Sa tu bajyabhyantarastambhavrittirdesakalasankhyabhi paridristwo dirghasuksma.***

The external wave, the internal wave and the straight wave are seen as long and subtle in space and time and number.

The following can be known personally from the *Guru*:

Drawing the air from the outside and trying to find the tranquil state at the end of exhaling which is the external sentiment (*bahira bhava*).

Trying to find the tranquil Breath at the end of inhaling, which is the internal sentiment (*antara bhava*).

The absence of straight and circular wave (*stambavriti bhava*).

### *51*

### ***Bajyabhyantara bisayakshepi chaturtha.***

From the viewpoint of analysis, the cessation of motion : apart from these three types of *Pranayam* which depend on external and internal waves and are indicated in space, time and number : is called the fourth *Pranayam*.

### *52*

### ***Tata kshiyate prakasabaranam.***

Later on, under the influence of Yoga practice, the obstructions to illumination are removed. Thereby all sufferings are removed.

### *53*

### ***Dharanasu cha yogyata manasa.***

By the practice of *Pranayam*, gradually a concept *Dharana*, or a true concept is formed.

## *54*

***Abisayasamprayoge chittvasya swarupanukara ibendriyanam pratyahara.***

In the absence of enjoyment of the Senses, that is, the absence of the application ml the eyes and tongue for seeing and tasting, the heart or *Chittva* then looks forward to being established in Tranquility. This is called *Pratyahara.*

## *55*

***Tata parama basyatendriyanam.***

Thereby the senses come under complete control.

# Chapter 3

# Bibhuti Pada : Powers

### *1*

### *Desabandhachittvasyadharana.*

Concept, or *Dharana* described after the first external five steps:

Breath ceases to flow when the waves of the heart concentrate at the lumbar center, the dorsal center, the inner Light at the *Kutastha*, the tip of the nose, the tip of the tongue or any external objects. This is called *Dharana*, or concept.

### *2*

### *Tatra pratyayoikatanata dhyanam.*

When the seeker continuously and undistractedly holds onto that Place (where true concept is held), this is called *Dhyana*, or meditation.

*3*

***Tadebarthamatranirbhasang Swarupasunyamiba samadhi.***

When the meditator (mind), the object of meditation (*Brahma*, the ultimate Sell) and meditation itself become one, beyond the awareness of the knowledge of meditation, only then will there be a Void like awareness which is called *Samadhi*, or Attunement.

*4*

***Trayamekatra sangjama.***

When these three : meditation, a glimpse of Tranquility and attunement : together become one, this is called *Sanjam*, or concentration.

*5*

***Tajjayat prajnaloka.***

Whoever masters this concentration becomes poised in the inner Light of Wisdom. Whenever he concentrates, he will receive inner Wisdom, that is, inner Realization.

*6*

***Tasya bhumisu biniyoga.***

The waves, or attachments, of the heart must be removed.

When the attachments of the heart are transcended, then the transcendental state is conquered.

Yoga provides knowledge of Yoga, and Yoga engages in Yoga, and when one is mad about Yoga, then he lives in Yoga.

*7*

***Trayamantarangang purbebhya.***

*Dhyana, Dharana* and *Samadhi* : respectively, meditation, concept, and attunement - are the inner Side towards *Sapragnat Samadhi*, or the unconsolidated state of *Samadhi*. The first five steps such as *Yama* and *Niyama* are external.

*8*

***Tadapi bahirangang nirbijasya.***

Even *Dhyana* and *Dharana*, that is, meditation and concept, are external to *Nirjiva*, or *Asampragnat Samadhi*, that is, to the state beyond *Omkar*, or inner Sound.

*9*

***Buthvana nirodhasangskarayorabhibhaba pradurbhaboi nirodhakshanachittvanayo nirodhaparinama.***

Appearance of the innate feeling is *Sanskara*. When and if *Sanskara* does appear, it is the sign of concentration and Tranquility of the heart, which is the result. Excitement of the wave, or attachment, of the heart is the nature of the heart.

Therefore, when the heart is tranquil by concentration, then there is no reappearance of *Sanskara*, or innate feelings.

Thus *Samadhi*, or attunement, is achieved.

***10***

***Tasya prasantabahita sangskarat.***

When the concentration of restraint is consolidated, then the feeling of reappearance of innate feelings is dissolved, and the heart becomes tranquil.

***11***

***Sarbathatoikagratayo kshayadao chittvasya samadhi parinama.***

Destruction of outwardness and generating the concentration of inwardness will result in *Samadhi*, or attunement.

***12***

***Santoditoi tulyapratayoi chittvasyaoikagrata parinam.***

Concentration finds the equilibrium state between Tranquility and reappearance of the *vrittis*, or waves.

### *13*

### *Etena bhutendriyesu dharmalakshanabastha parinam byakhyata.*

The character, definition and state of five elements and the ten sense organs are known by concentration. For example, the characteristic of mud is changed into something else when the clay pot is baked at a high temperature.

Similarly, the nature and various states of the sense organs are also known.

### *14*

### *Tatra santoditabyapadesya dharmanupati dharmi.*

According to the manifestation of the waves of the heart, such as tranquility, excitement and non pervasiveness (the area not fit for pervasion), the unceasing power of cause and effect is called character.

Manifestation takes its character according to its nature.

The ring of the hand and the ring of the ear are both made of gold, but the apparent manifestation differs. By seeing the apparent manifestation, one can understand its nature.

### *15*

### *Kramanyattvang parinamanyatve hetu.*

How are different states of manifestation made possible from the same one substance?

The different states are the cause of the different states of manifestation.

By that knowledge of different gradation, the manifestation of *Brahma*, the ultimate Self is proven.

### *16*

### *Parinamatraya sangjamadatiianagatajnanam.*

By concentration on these three categories of manifestation : namely, character, definition and different states : knowledge of the past and future is attained.

### *17*

### *Sabdartha pratyayanamitaretaradhyasang sankarastat prabibhaga sangjamat sarbabhutarutajnanam.*

By concentration on sound, meaning and vibration and the transcendence of reason, knowledge of this mixture is acquired.

If one concentrates separately on each division, then the meaning of sound of all beings is attained.

In the utterance of happiness or suffering of all animals, there is similarity.

*18*

***Sanskara sakshatkaranang purbajatijnanam.***

The present life comes into manifestation due to innate feelings of the past lives called *Sanskara.*

Through concentration one can comc to know from which class a man or other living beings has come into present manifestation.

*19*

***Pratayasya parachittvajnanam.***

By concentration on notion (vibration), the knowledge of others' hearts is known.

*20*

***Na cha tasyalambanang tasyabisayi bhutatvat.***

With the knowledge of others' hearts, the knowledge of the objects of others' hearts is not possible to know because this is outside the field of concentration.

*21*

***Kayarupasangjamat tadagrajyasaktistambhe chakshu prakasamprayoge yantardhanam.***

By concentration on the body, the Yogi can keep away from the sight of others who cannot see him due to high vibration.

*22*

***Eten sabdadyantardhanamuktam.***

In this case, even sound is included. That is, by this process, a Yogi can make sounds which will be unheard by others.

*23*

***Sopakramannirupakramancha karma tat sangjamada parantajnanam aristobhyo ba.***

There are two kinds of action:

1. Those with expectation for results therefrom and

2. Those without expectation for results.

By the power of concentration on action, the event called death and all spiritual and material events and their relevant circumstances are known. Birth, decay and death, etc., are the results of actions.

By the influence of concentration, even the knowledge of future results of actions is attained.

*24*

***Moitradisu balani.***

By friendship and kindness, strength is generated.

25

***Balesu hastibaladini.***

By concentration on the strength of the elephant, strength is attained.

26

***Pravittyalokanyasat suksmabyabhita biprakristajnanam.***

By concentration on the illuminating character of the mind and on what was told before, subtle things situated at a distance or things in far places can be known.

27

***Bhuabanajnanang surya sangjamat.***

If one concentrates on the Sun, then knowledge of the seven worlds is attained.

28

***Chandre tarabyuhajnanam.***

By concentration on the moon, knowledge of the stars are attained.

29

***Dhrube tadgatijnanam.***

Concentrating on the Pole Star, knowledge of the speed of the stars is acquired.

*30*

***Navichakre kayabyuhajnanam.***

By concentration on the lumber center, knowledge of the physical body is achieved.

*31*

***Kanthakupe kshutpipasanivrittvi.***

When concentration is fixed on the throat, hunger is satisfied.

*32*

***Kumanadyang sthaoirjyam.***

By concentration on the *Kurma* nerve, the seeker can calm the mind.

*33*

***Murdha jyotisi siddha darsanam.***

By concentration on the inner Light between the eyebrows by *Yonimudra* practice, the Yogi can see the *Siddhas*, or the realized Ones of the past.

*34*

***Pratibhadba sarbam.***

By concentration on Venus, all knowledge is attained.

*35*

***Hridaye chittva sangbit.***

By concentration on the dorsal center, knowledge of the heart is achieved.

### *36*

***Satva purusayortyantasangkirnayo pratyayabisesabhoga parathatvang swarthasangjamat purisajnanam.***

Enjoyment is defined as unspecific impressions of the person, or *Purusa.* There is a difference between consciousness and unconsciousness and between enjoyment and the object of enjoyment on the part of *Purusa* and the *Sattva* (the doctrine of intelligence).

This is a different form of Realization.

Separate from this different form of Realization, by concentrating only on the form of Purusa (only by the knowledge of the ultimate Self), the knowledge of the *Purusa*, or person, is attained.

### *37*

***Tara pratibha sravanabedanadarsawadavarta jayante.***

By concentration, the knowledge of Venus (that is, the knowledge of subtleties), distance, arrangements, past and unwelcome knowledge, divine Sound, touch, vision and taste are attained.

### *38*

***Te samadhabupasarga byuthane siddhaya.***

All the aforesaid yogic powers are obstructions to attaining *Samadhi*, or attunement (with the ultimate Self), although they are effective in bringing fruits to the practical life.

### *39*

***Bandhakaranasoithilang pracharasangbedanachha chittvasya parasarira besa.***

When the breath is tranquil, the past deposits of actions, which are the cause of the restlessness of the heart, become loose.

Due to the expansion of heart into another's body, the Yogi can enter another's body and the senses follow the mind.

### *40*

***Udanajayajjwalapankajantakadisvasanga utkrantischa.***

When the Yogi masters *Udana Bayu* (breath), which operates at the throat center, then due to the Tranquil Breath of the upper side and the Tranquil Breath of the lower side, the body of the Yogi becomes light. Water, mud and thorns cannot touch his body, which is raised above these things.

### *41*

***Samana jayajjwalanam.***

When the Yogi masters *Saman Bayu*, that is, the breath operating at the lumbar center, then due to the putting down (lowering) of the energy of the upper side to the lower side, he becomes like fire.

***42***
***Srotrakasayo sambandhasangjamadibyasrotram.***

By concentration on the relation between the sky and the hearing organ, the power of divine Hearing and subtle distance is known. Subtle sound and sky and hearing are sensible.

***43***
***Kayakasayo sambandha sanjamal Iughutula samaptteschа akasagamanam.***

By concentration on the relation between the body and the sky, the body becomes as light as cotton and moves in the sky.

***44***
***Bahiraklpitavrittvir mahabidehattvat prakas abarana kshaya.***

Outward awareness, due to outward attention and egoism, is imagination. Outward awareness without egoism is lack of imagination, that is, neutral.

By concentration on the great disembodiment, the curtain of revelation is destroyed. All impurities are destroyed.

### 45

### *Sthulaswarupasuksmanwayarthabatva sangjamad bhuta jaya.*

Beings come under control through concentration on these five things: gross elements, forms, subtleties, analysis and meaning.

The manifested forms of beings are the gross forms of the five elements:

1. Thinness, warmth, etc.
2. Subtle forms of smell, etc., due to a variation of causes.
3. The all-pervading illuminating tendency which comes from tranquility.
4. Meaning, which is the power of performance for the enjoyment of those qualities.
5. Concentration on the quality of beings, which may be brought under the control of the Yogi in any form.

### 46

### *Tato animadi pradurbhaba kayasampattardharmmanabhi ghatascha.*

Afterwards, the influence of *Anima*, etc., begins.

1. *Anima*, that is, becoming small as one sees a small star everywhere, gradually moving here and there unnoticed.

2. *Laghima*: Becoming light;
3. *Mahima*: Becoming large; the power of touching the moon, etc.
4. *Prapti*: Getting everything;
5. *Prakamya*: (Being) satisfied;
6. *Isitwa*: Like the Lord;
7. *Basitwa*: Control; and
8. *Kamyabasayita*: Mastery over desires.

These eightfold yogic powers, the physical aspect and transitoriness of the body bringing all things under control, such fearlessness from fire and water, etc., and moving in space : all these powers are acquired.

### 47

***Rupalabanyabalabraja sanghananatvani kayasampat.***

The following are attained: handsomeness, loveliness, strength and the power for bearing hardship.

### 48

***Grahana swaruoasmitanvayarthabattva sangjamadindriya jaya.***

By concentration on the functions of the senses, form, egoism, relation and meaning, the power for controlling the senses is attained.

*49*

***Tatomanojabitvang bikaranabhaba pradhana jayascha.***

Thereby, one acquires speed like the mind and wins the influence of Nature's manifestation.

*50*

***Satva purusanyatakhyati matrasya sarbabhab adhisthatritang sarbajnatritancha.***

When knowledge about substance and Person arises, one can keep all beings under control and acquire omniscience.

*51*

***Tadwoiragyadapi dosabijalshaye kaibalyam.***

Wheat the spirit of renunciation is generated in that state of Consciousness, then the seed of attachment is destroyed and the state of *Kaibalya*, that is, eternal Realization, is achieved.

*62*

***Sthanupyanimantrane sangasmayakaranang punaranista prasangagat.***

The Yogi should not be attached to nor surprised if some mysterious sound and/or things come before him.

Although *Brahma* is eternally Tranquil in the Atom, yet the mind under the senses again tries to do harm by going outward.

Hence, being tempted, the Yogi must not exhibit yogic powers.

### *53*

***Kshanatatkramayo sangjamadvivekajang jnanam.***

If concentration is on the moment (atom of time) and its state of *before* and *after* the intellect is dissolved, Realization starts.

When one is eternally established in *Brahma*, the ultimate Self, and in the subtle form of the Star, then Knowledge or Realization begins.

### *54*

***Jatilakshanadesoiranyatan abachhedattulyayostata pratipattvi.***

In the absence of caste, signs, nations (places), etc., opposite things become the same.

### *55*

***Tarakang sarbabisayang sarbatha bisayamkramancheti tad vivekajang jnanam.***

Absolute Knowledge and all relative knowledge are due to inner Realization.

When the subtle Star is eternally known everywhere, then inner Realization is achieved.

### *56*

***Sattva purusayo suddhisamye kaibalyam.***

The universal, or infinite, state of pure Consciousness of the ultimate Self is the state of *Kaibalya.*

# Chapter 4

# Kaivalya Pada : Realization : Sthirattva (Eternal Tranquility)

*1*

***Janmosadhi mantratapa samadhija siddhaya.***

One can attain powers even under the influence of a past life, medicine. *Mantras* (the chanting of syllables), *tapasya* (austerities), *Samadhi* (attunement).

*2*

***Tatrakayendriyanamanyajatiya parinatanam jatyastara parinam prakrityapurat.***

What the reason is for the influence of past lives is described as follows:

According to the influence of nature, one category of body and the senses becomes different, that is, the senses take shape according to inner feelings.

Therefore, the attainments of previous lives automatically accrue in the next life.

*3*

***Nimittam prayojakam prakritanam varanabhedastu tata kshetrikabat.***

Religion is not the cause of the instigation of all sorts of natures. When the veil of concealment is removed, that is, when obstruction is destroyed, nature is able to work accordingly.

As the owner of the land shall not have any difficulty in bringing water to his land from some other piece of land when the barrier between them is destroyed and water automatically flows there, likewise, when the veil of obstruction of religion and non-religion is removed, the intellect passes from one body to another. The attainment of godliness by *Nandikeswar* and the concept of King *Nahus* becoming a kingsnake are examples thereof.

*4*

***Nimanachittvanyasmitamatrat.***

Intellectual speculation results in the manifold nature of heart.

*5*

***Pravrittvibhede prayojakang chittvamekamanekoisam.***

According to the different nature of speculations, the heart of those manifold speculations is the same.

*6*

***Tatra dhyanajamanasayam.***

The contemplative heart, being free from action and results, is greater than any other kind, due to the influence of previous lifetimes in five different ways.

*7*

***Karmasuklakrisnang yoginastribidhimitaresam.***

Actions are of four kinds:

1. White: honest, as the making of donations or practice of austerities.
2. Black: dishonest.
3. Black and white: outwardly honest, but in fact, inflicting injuries upon others.
4. The performance of actions without expecting any results therefrom, whether good or bad.

Among these four types of actions, the Yogi is engaged in the last one and ordinary people are engaged in the first three.

### *8*

***Tatastadwipakanu gunanamebabhibyakti vasananam.***

Due to the first three above-mentioned types of actions, desires manifest accordingly.

### *9*

***Jatidesakal byabahitanamapyanantarjyang smriti sangskarayoreka rupatvat.***

Resemblance remains even after the great difference that exists between castes, nations, and time, due to the permanent form of remembrance.

Innate feelings/tendencies of many previous lives share similarities.

### *10*

***Tasamanadityang chasiso nityatvat.***

Those desires are beginningless, as blessings, that is, the desire for welfare is always present.

### *11*

***Hetu phalasrayalambanoi sanggritatvadesambhabe tadbhaba.***

Desires are accumulated due to causes, and the accumulation of effects and causes give rise to sentiment.

If there are no causes and accumulations or results (effects), then there are no desires. Due to the absence of a particular cause, a particular desire is dissolved.

### *12*

***Atitanagatang swarupatoyastyadhvabhedamarmanam.***

Due to the Realization of true Religion, the past and future are present in actuality.

### *13*

***Te byaktasukshma gunatmana.***

Those manifested and subtle things are qualified, that is, their substance is under the qualities

### *14*

***Parinamoikattvadwastutattvam.***

Things are due to one state of manifestation. Finally, all things automatically become One.

### *15*

***Bastusamye chittabhedattayorbibikta pantha.***

There are different ways of knowledge and meaning concerning the same thing due to the difference of heart.

The One Self is everywhere; due to the absence of Realization, the sense of discrimination is there.

### *16*

***Tradu paragapekshitvachhittvasya bastujnatajnatam.***

The knowledge of objects is in the heart in proportion to attachment to that particular object.

All objects are in one rhythm in the heart, but they are not the true rhythm of *Brahma*, the ultimate Self. When this is understood, then knowledge of an object is gained in proportion to the attachment to that object.

### *17*

***Sadajnataschittvavrittayastat prabho purusasya parinamitvat.***

Since the supreme Person of the heart had no indisposition, all the waves of the heart were already known.

### *18*

***Na tat swabhasang drisyatat.***

*That* is not radiant because of seeing. The radiant Self is not seen by ordinary eyes but can be known by the grace of the *Guru*.

*19*

***Ek samaye chobhayanabadharanam.***

It is not possible to attain the knowledge of *Brahma* and the knowledge of objects at the same time.

*20*

***Chittvantaradrisye buddhibuddherati prasanga smriti sankarascha.***

If the intellect is known by another intellect, then for that other intellect, again another intellect is needed. Thus intellect ad infinitum is necessary, and there is a mixture of remembrance. When the Self is realized in all things, then the intellect can be tranquil.

*21*

***Kathang chitcra pratisangkramayastadakarapatto swa buddhi sangbedanam.***

When the ever-stationed supreme Being becomes One with the waves of the intellect, the vibration of the intellect starts.

In spite of the physical form, the Atom of *Brahma*, the ultimate Self, is within and without.

The form of things is the ultimate Self, that is, *Brahma* or the ultimate self is possible only in things.

*22*

***Drasta drisyoparaktang chittvang sarbartham.***

Becoming One with the seer and the manifestation of the receiver of the seen are the objects of the heart.

Both seer and seen, that is, the subject and the object, are *Brahma.*

Therefore, by knowledge of the same, omniscience is achieved.

*23*

***Tadasangkhyeya vasanabhischittvamapi pararthang sanghatyakaritvat.***

The heart is full of desires which are unitedly effective, meant for *Brahma.*

Both the hearts filled with unlimited desires and the individuals who are desiring are actually One, the ultimate Self, *Brahma.*

*24*

***Bisesadarsina atmabhaba bhabana nivrittvi.***

Egoism is dissolved in the Yogi who has come to realize the supreme Being. The feeling of doership and attachment is dissolved in the realized Yogi.

### 25

***Tadavivekanimnang kaibalya pragabharang chittvam.***

Then, the ignorant heart, which is full of attachment awareness of knowledge, moves toward the state of *Kaibalya*, that is, to be blessed by the *Guru*'s grace.

### 26

***Tachhidresu pratyayantarani sangskarebhya.***

Due to previous innate feelings, even in the background of *Kaibalya* notions arise.

### 27

***Hanamesang klesubaduktam.***

These innate feelings must be destroyed by means previously described for the destruction of ignorance.

### 28

***Prasangkhyaneyapyakusidasya sarbathaviveka khyate dharmamegha samadhi.***

*Dharmamegha Samadhi* is attained due to knowledge accrued from the practice of Kriya abandoning the results therefrom.

*29*

***Tata klesakarmanitrittvi.***

Then actions and suffering due to ignorance are dissolved.

*30*

***Tadasarbaranamalapetasya jnanasyang jneyamalpam.***

Then all obstructions and limitations are destroyed due to Knowledge; therefore nothing remains to be known any longer.

*31*

***Tata kritarthanamparinamakramasamaptir gunanam.***

Then the different states of divine qualities of the realized Person are transcended.

*32*

***Kshanapratiyogi parinamaparanta nigrajya krama.***

At the time of transcending the state of manifestation which may be momentur the Star of Consciousness between the eyebrows will always be seen.

*33*

***Purusarthasunyanang gunanampratì prasaba kaibalyang swarupa pratistha ba chitisaktiriti.***

*Kaibalya* is the transcendence of attachment and egoism, the manifestation of the reverse order of qualities and being established in Consciousness, remaining only in that state. When the heart is tranquil by the practice of *Pranayam*, or Kriya, and by the transcendence of qualities, the inner Self will automatically establish himself in Oneness with the ultimate Self. This is the state of *Kaibalya.*

***OM Shanti ! Shanti !! Shanti !!!***

ॐ

# LIST OF TITLES WITH ISBN NO.

| ISBN | TITLE |
|---|---|
| 9788194914129 | 1984 |
| 9789390575220 | 1984 & Animal Farm (2In1) |
| 9789390575572 | 1984 & Animal Farm (2In1): The International Best-Selling Classics |
| 9789390575848 | 35 Sonnets |
| 9789390575329 | A Clergyman's Daughter |
| 9789390575923 | A Study In Scarlet |
| 9789390896097 | A Tale Of Two Cities |
| 9789390896837 | Abide in Christ |
| 9789390896202 | Abraham Lincoln |
| 9789390896912 | Absolute Surrender |
| 9789390896608 | African American Classic Collection |
| 9789390575305 | Aldous Huxley: The Collected Works |
| 9789390896141 | An Autobiography of M. K. Gandhi |
| 9789390575886 | Animal Farm |
| 9789390575619 | Animal Farm & The Great Gatsby (2In1) |
| 9789390575626 | Animal Farm & We |
| 9789390896158 | Anna Karenina |
| 9789390575534 | Antic Hay |
| 9789390896165 | Antony & Cleopatra |
| 9789390896172 | As I Lay Dying |
| 9789390896226 | As You like it |
| 9789390575671 | At Your Command |
| 9789390575350 | Awakened Imagination |
| 9789390575114 | Be What You Wish |
| 9789390896233 | Believe In yourself |
| 9789390896998 | Best of Charles Darwin: The Origin of Species & Autobiography |
| 9789390896684 | Best Of Horror : Dracula And Frankenstein |
| 9789390575503 | Best Of Mark Twain (The Adventures of Tom Sawyer AND The Adventures of Huckleberry Finn) |
| 9789390896769 | Black History Collection |
| 9789390575756 | Brave New World, Animal Farm & 1984 (3in1) |

| | |
|---|---|
| 9789390896240 | Brother Karamzov |
| 9789390575053 | Bulleh Shah Poetry |
| 9789390575725 | Burmese Days |
| 9789390896257 | Bushido |
| 9789390896066 | Can't Hurt Me |
| 9788194914112 | Chanakya Neeti: With The Complete Sutras |
| 9789390896042 | Crime and Punishment |
| 9789390575527 | Crome Yellow |
| 9789390575046 | Down and Out in Paris and London |
| 9789390896844 | Dracula |
| 9789390575442 | Emersons Essays: The Complete First & Second Series (Self-Reliance & Other Essays) |
| 9789390575749 | Emma |
| 9789390575817 | Essential Tozer Collection - The Pursuit of God & The Purpose of Man |
| 9789390896578 | Fascism What It Is and How to Fight It |
| 9789390575688 | Feeling is the Secret |
| 9789390575190 | Five Lessons |
| 9789390575954 | Frankenstein |
| 9789390575237 | Franz Kafka: Collected Works |
| 9789390575282 | Franz Kafka: Short Stories |
| 9789390575060 | George Orwell Collected Works |
| 9789390575077 | George Orwell Essays |
| 9789390575213 | George Orwell Poems |
| 9788194914150 | Greatest Poetry Ever Written Vol 1 |
| 9788194914143 | Greatest Poetry Ever Written Vol 1 |
| 9789390896301 | Gulliver's Travel |
| 9789390575961 | Gunaho Ka Devta |
| 9789390575893 | H. P. Lovecraft Selected Stories Vol 1 |
| 9789390575978 | H. P. Lovecraft Selected Stories Vol 2 |
| 9789390896059 | Hamlet |
| 9789390575022 | His Last Bow: Some Reminiscences of Sherlock Holmes |
| 9789390896134 | History of Western Philosophy |
| 9789390575121 | Homage To Catalonia |

| | |
|---|---|
| 9789390896219 | How to develop self-confidence and Improve public Speaking |
| 9789390896295 | How to enjoy your life and your Job |
| 9789390575633 | How to own your own mind |
| 9789390896318 | How to read Human Nature |
| 9789390896325 | How to sell your way through the life |
| 9789390896370 | How to use the laws of mind |
| 9789390896387 | How to use the power of prayer |
| 9789390896028 | How to win friends & Influence People |
| 9788194824176 | How To Win Friends and Influence People |
| 9789390896103 | Humility The Beauty of Holiness |
| 9789390896653 | Imperialism the Highest Stage of Capitalism |
| 9789390575084 | In Our Time |
| 9789390575169 | In Our Time & Three Stories and Ten poems |
| 9789390575145 | James Allen: The Collected Works |
| 9789390896189 | Jesus Himself |
| 9789390575480 | Jo's Boys |
| 9789390896394 | Julius Caesar |
| 9789390575404 | Keep the Aspidistra Flying |
| 9789390896400 | Kidnapped |
| 9789390896424 | King Lear |
| 9789390575824 | Lady Susan |
| 9789390896455 | Law of Success |
| 9789390896264 | Lincoln The Unknown |
| 9789390575565 | Little Men |
| 9789390575640 | Little Women |
| 9788194914174 | Lost Horizon |
| 9789390896462 | Macbeth |
| 9789390896929 | Man Eaters of Kumaon |
| 9789390896523 | Man The Dwelling Place of God |
| 9789390896349 | Man The Dwelling Place of God |
| 9789390575909 | Mansfield Park |
| 9788194914136 | Manto Ki 25 Sarvshreshth Kahaniya |
| 9789390896509 | Marxism, Anarchism, Communism |
| 9789390575664 | Mathematical Principles of Natural Philosophy |

| | |
|---|---|
| 9788194914198 | Meditations |
| 9789390575800 | Mein Kampf |
| 9789390575794 | Memory How To Develop, Train, And Use It |
| 9789390896486 | Mind Power |
| 9789390896585 | Money |
| 9789390575039 | Mortal Coils |
| 9789390575770 | My Life and Work |
| 9789390896035 | Narrative of the Life of Frederick Douglass |
| 9789390575152 | Neville Goddard: The Collected Works |
| 9789390575985 | Northanger Abbey |
| 9789390896530 | Notes From Underground |
| 9789390896547 | Oliver Twist |
| 9789390575459 | On War |
| 9789390575541 | One, None and a Hundred Thousand |
| 9789390896554 | Othelo |
| 9789390575435 | Out Of This World |
| 9789390575015 | Persuasion |
| 9789390575510 | Prayer The Art Of Believing |
| 9789390575091 | Pride and Prejudice |
| 9789390896561 | Psychic Perception |
| 9789390575381 | Rabindranath Tagore - 5 Best Short Stories Vol 2 |
| 9789390575367 | Rabindranath Tagore - Short Stories (Masters Collections Including The Childs Return) |
| 9789390575374 | Rabindranath Tagore 5 Best Short Stories Vol 1 (Including The Childs Return |
| 9789390896622 | Romeo & Juliet |
| 9789390896127 | Sanatana Dharma |
| 9789390575596 | Seedtime & Harvest |
| 9789390896639 | Selected Stories of Guy De Maupassant |
| 9789390575206 | Self-Reliance & Other Essays |
| 9789390575176 | Sense and Sensibility |
| 9789390575299 | Shyamchi Aai |
| 9789390896738 | Socialism Utopian and Scientific |
| 9789390896646 | Success Through a Positive Mental Attitude |
| 9789390575428 | The Adventures of Huckleberry Finn |

| | |
|---|---|
| 9789390575183 | The Adventures of Sherlock Holmes |
| 9789390575343 | The Adventures of Tom Sawyer |
| 9789390896691 | The Alchemy Of Happiness |
| 9789390575862 | The Art Of Public Speaking |
| 9789390896288 | The Autobiography Of Charles Darwin |
| 9788194914181 | The Best of Franz Kafka: The Metamorphosis & The Trial |
| 9789390575008 | The Call Of Cthulhu and Other Weird Tales |
| 9789390575107 | The Case-Book of Sherlock Holmes |
| 9789390896110 | The Castle Of Otranto |
| 9789390896745 | The Communist Manifesto |
| 9789390575589 | The Complete Fiction of H. P. Lovecraft |
| 9789390575497 | The Complete Works of Florence Scovel Shinn |
| 9789390896820 | The Conquest of Breard |
| 9789390896813 | The Diary of a Young Girl |
| 9789390896332 | The Diary of a Young Girl The Definitive Edition of the Worlds Most Famous Diary |
| 9789390575701 | The Great Gatsby, Animal Farm & 1984 (3In1) |
| 9789390575312 | The Greatest Works Of George Orwell (5 Books) Including 1984 & Non-Fiction |
| 9789390575992 | The Hound of Baskervilles |
| 9789390896707 | The Idiot |
| 9789390896714 | The Invisible Man |
| 9789390575657 | The Knowledge of the holy |
| 9789390575558 | The Law & the Promise |
| 9789390896721 | The Law Of Attraction |
| 9789390896776 | The Leader in you |
| 9789390896363 | The Life of Christ |
| 9789390896196 | The Man-Eating Leopard of Rudraprayag |
| 9789390896783 | The Master Key to Riches |
| 9789390575268 | The Memoirs Of Sherlock Holmes |
| 9789390896479 | The Midsummer Night's Dream |
| 9789390575466 | The Mill On The Floss |
| 9789390896790 | The Miracles of your mind |
| 9789390896660 | The Mutual Aid A Factor in Evolution |
| 9789390896448 | The Origin of Species |

| | |
|---|---|
| 9789390896905 | The Peter Kropotkin Anthology The Conquest of Bread & Mutual Aid A Factor of Evolution |
| 9789390896806 | The Picture of Dorian Gray |
| 9789390896271 | The Picture of Dorian Gray |
| 9789390575275 | The Power Of Awareness |
| 9789390896356 | The Power of Concentration |
| 9788194824169 | The Power of Positive Thinking |
| 9789390575411 | The Power of the Spoken Word |
| 9788194914105 | The Power Of Your Subconscious Mind |
| 9789390896899 | The Power of Your Subconscious Mind |
| 9789390896417 | The Principles of Communism |
| 9789390575787 | The Psychology Of Mans Possible Evolution |
| 9789390896615 | The Psychology of Salesmanship |
| 9789390575732 | The Pursuit of God |
| 9789390575398 | The Pursuit of Happiness |
| 9789390896851 | The Quick and Easy Way to effective Speaking |
| 9789390575947 | The Return Of Sherlock Holmes |
| 9789390575138 | The Road To Wigan Pier |
| 9789390896981 | The Root of the Righteous |
| 9789390575855 | The Science Of Being Well |
| 9788194914167 | The Science Of Getting Rich, The Science Of Being Great & The Science Of Being Well (3In1) |
| 9789390896011 | The Screwtape Letters |
| 9789390896073 | The Screwtape Letters |
| 9789390575336 | The Secret Door to Success |
| 9789390575695 | The Secret Of Imagining |
| 9789390896868 | The Secret Of Success |
| 9789390896431 | The Seven Last Words |
| 9789390575930 | The Sign of the Four |
| 9789390896004 | The Sonnets |
| 9789390896516 | The Souls of Black Folk |
| 9789390896875 | The Sound and The Fury |
| 9789390575244 | The State and Revolution |
| 9789390896882 | The Story of My Life |
| 9789390896936 | The Story Of Oriental Philosophy |

| | |
|---|---|
| 9789390896752 | The Strange Case of Dr. Jekyll and Mr. Hyde |
| 9789390896943 | The Tempest |
| 9789390575916 | The Valley Of Fear |
| 9789390575879 | The Wind in the willows |
| 9789390896080 | The Wind in the willows |
| 9789390575763 | Their eyes were watching gofd |
| 9789390575831 | Three Stories |
| 9789390896950 | Twelfth Night |
| 9789390896592 | Twelve Years a Slave |
| 9789390896677 | Up from Slavery |
| 9789390896974 | Value Price and Profit |
| 9789390896967 | Wake Up and Live |
| 9789390896493 | With Christ in the School of Prayer |
| 9789390575602 | Your Faith is Your Fortune |
| 9789390575473 | Your Infinite Power To Be Rich |
| 9789390575251 | Your Word is Your Wand |
| 9789390575718 | Youth |
| 9789391316099 | A Christmas Carol |
| 9789391316105 | A Doll's House |
| 9789391316501 | A Passage to India |
| 9789391316709 | A Portrait of the Artist as a Young Man |
| 9789391316112 | A Tale of Two Cities |
| 9789391316747 | A Tear and a Smile |
| 9789391316167 | Agnes Gray |
| 9789391316174 | Alice's Adventures in Wonderland |
| 9789391316136 | Anandamath |
| 9789391316181 | Anne Of Green Gables |
| 9789391316754 | Anthem |
| 9789391316198 | Around The World in 80 Days |
| 9789391316013 | As A Man Thinketh |
| 9789391316242 | Autobiography of a Yogi |
| 9789391316266 | Beyond Good and Evil |
| 9789391316761 | Bleak House |
| 9789391316778 | Chitra, a Play in One Act |
| 9789391316310 | David Copperfield |

| | |
|---|---|
| 9789391316075 | Demian |
| 9789391316785 | Dubliners |
| 9789391316051 | Favourite Tales from the Arabian Nights |
| 9789391316235 | Gitanjali |
| 9789391316068 | Gravity |
| 9789391316150 | Great Speeches of Abraham Lincoln |
| 9789391316662 | Guerilla Warfare |
| 9789391316839 | Kim |
| 9789391316822 | Mother |
| 9789391316211 | My Childhood |
| 9789391316846 | Nationalism |
| 9789391316327 | Oliver Twist |
| 9789391316853 | Pygmalion |
| 9789391316334 | Relativity: The Special and the General Theory |
| 9789391316389 | Scientific Healing Affirmation |
| 9789391316341 | Sons and Lovers |
| 9789391316587 | Tales from India |
| 9789391316372 | Tess of The D'Urbervilles |
| 9789391316396 | The Awakening and Selected Stories |
| 9789391316402 | The Bhagvad Gita |
| 9789391316303 | The Book of Enoch |
| 9789391316228 | The Canterville Ghost |
| 9789391316907 | The Dynamic Laws of Prosperity |
| 9789391316006 | The Great Gatsby |
| 9789391316860 | The Hungry Stones and Other Stories |
| 9789391316433 | The Idiot |
| 9789391316440 | The Importance of Being Earnest |
| 9789391316297 | The Light of Asia |
| 9789391316914 | The Madman His Parables and Poems |
| 9789391316457 | The Odyssey |
| 9789391316921 | The Picture of Dorian Gray |
| 9789391316464 | The Prince |
| 9789391316938 | The Prophet |
| 9789391316945 | The Republic |
| 9789391316518 | The Scarlet Letter |

| | |
|---|---|
| 9789391316143 | The Seven Laws of Teaching |
| 9789391316525 | The Story of My Experiments with Truth |
| 9789391316532 | The Tales of the Mother Goose |
| 9789391316549 | The Thirty Nine Steps |
| 9789391316594 | The Time Machine |
| 9789391316600 | The Turn of the Screw |
| 9789391316983 | The Upanishads |
| 9789391316617 | The Yellow Wallpaper |
| 9789391316426 | The Yoga Sutras of Patanjali |
| 9789391316990 | Ulysses |
| 9789391316624 | Utopia |
| 9789391316679 | Vanity Fair |
| 9789391316020 | What Is To Be Done |
| 9789391316686 | Within A Budding Grove |
| 9789391316693 | Women in Love |